The Meno

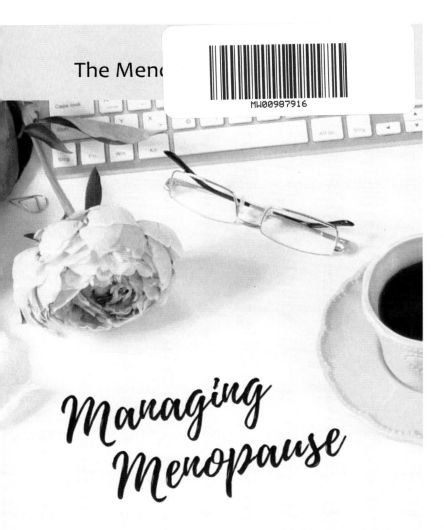

Managing Menopause

THE ULTIMATE MENOPAUSE GUIDEBOOK

DR. MICHELLE GORDON

Year of the Book
135 Glen Avenue
Glen Rock, PA 17327

Print ISBN: 978-1-949150-58-2
Ebook ISBN: 978-1-949150-59-9

Contents

Foreword

What Is Menopause?

Menopause is more than just the end of our child-bearing years. Menopause is a journey—one for which many of us arrive unprepared and surprised.

We often wonder what's happening to us, why our faces intermittently feel like they're on fire, and why our moods bounce from one extreme to another. The symptoms of menopause can be life-changing. We gain weight, or stop wanting to be sexually active. Sleep disturbances upset our daily lives, and we are often left feeling tired and worn down. Anxiety may rear its ugly head and we don't know how to interact due to crippling fear. Not to mention the brain fog that makes us lose our keys, phone, or double-book appointments... sometimes resulting in fractured relationships.

Why is menopause such a big secret? Why is it that every single woman goes through it, but yet it seems like no one is talking about it? It could be the media's constant glorification of youth. It could be that women in the past just managed and didn't talk about it.

In this book we remove the veil of secrecy around menopause. We talk about the physiology, the psychology, and what it all means. We address many of the symptoms and possible treatments. We also intersperse anecdotes and stories from menopausal women.

We hope you enjoy this book, and we look forward to seeing you in our Facebook community at http://www.facebook.com/groups/menopausemovement

Menopause

Menopause is when a woman's periods stop and she is no longer fertile. The average age of menopause is about 51 years but it can occur anywhere from age 40 to 59. Menopause is usually preceded by "perimenopause" for a few years.

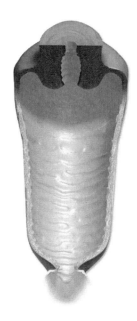

MENOPAUSE

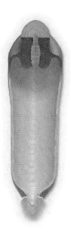

In perimenopause, the levels of estrogen and progesterone produced by the ovaries begin to decrease. The periods become irregular but do not stop altogether. Women can get symptoms of menopause during perimenopause (hot flashes, night sweats, and mood changes, to name a few) but they aren't as frequent as when a woman reaches menopause. A woman in perimenopause can get pregnant (often called a "change of life baby").

Premature Menopause

Premature menopause (ovarian failure) occurs in 1% of women. [1] It can be caused by genetics, auto-immune issues, surgery (removing the ovaries), viral infections, and/or toxic exposure.

It is sometimes referred to as premature ovarian failure or primary ovarian insufficiency. The ovaries are either absent (surgery) or stop producing hormones. This can result in early infertility.

The term "premature menopause" is often used interchangeably with premature ovarian failure but they are not exactly the same thing.

Women in premature menopause stop having periods prior to age 40, while women with premature ovarian failure may still ovulate, causing irregular periods. The treatment of premature ovarian failure

---

[1] Deepti Goswami, Gerard S. Conway; Premature ovarian failure, *Human Reproduction Update*, Volume 11, Issue 4, 1 July 2005, Pages 391–410, https://doi.org/10.1093/humupd/dmi012

is estrogen replacement therapy. This treats the symptoms but does not address infertility.

1 | The Three Stages of Menopause

There are actually three stages a woman goes through as part of the menopausal process. These are:

Perimenopause. The ovaries begin to decrease production of estrogen. There will be some symptoms of hot flashes and other menopausal symptoms but the woman will have occasional periods. Mood swings are common in perimenopause. Many women enter perimenopause sometime in their 40s while other women do not experience this stage at all.

> *Cindy was only 45, the youngest member of her book club, but when she started fanning herself with the current read, all the other women nodded knowingly.*
> *"Welcome to the club, Cindy!"*

Menopause. The periods finally stop. The woman is said to be in menopause when she has not had a period for at least 12 months. There are often symptoms, including mood swings, hot flashes, and night sweats. Menopause can last for 1-3 years.

> *Angela woke up at 3:00 am for the third time that week, bathed in a pool of sweat. She shoved off the covers, trudged to the bathroom (again), and opened the window on her way. She was freezing when she returned to bed.*

Post-menopause. The periods have finally stopped and the ovaries are no longer producing much estrogen at all. Usually the symptoms taper off but many women continue to have dry vaginal mucosa and are at an increased risk for osteoporosis and heart disease.

> *Gloria didn't miss the hot flashes, but her husband sure missed the days of romance without stopping to apply the extra lubricant.*

2 | Symptoms Of Perimenopause

As mentioned, some women will not have any symptoms in perimenopause, while others will have noticeable symptoms. Common symptoms of perimenopause include the following:

Hot flashes and night sweats. These are feelings of increased bodily warmth and flushing of the face. They can occur at any time of the day or night and can be uncomfortable. If they happen at night, the woman can experience night sweats, like Angela above.

Irregular periods. The ovaries may still ovulate but they do so in no predictable pattern. This can result in periods that are shorter than normal or periods that are longer than normal. The menstrual flow may be very heavy, especially if the period is short. Sometimes periods are skipped altogether, causing the woman to worry that she might be pregnant.

> *Ginny was noticing the hot flashes, but was so happy she didn't have a period. Then her clothes weren't fitting correctly. When the nausea*

> *and breast pain came, she couldn't*
> *believe it. Was it true? She sat*
> *dumbfounded in the bathroom*
> *looking at a positive pregnancy*
> *test. Her youngest, Billy, was 11! "I*
> *guess it's not menopause," she said*
> *to herself.*

Mood swings. Some women in perimenopause will suffer from an increased risk of depression or irritability during this stage. Sleep may be elusive as night sweats and hot flashes can happen during the night.

> *"I can't keep up with your mood*
> *swings, Mom!" Candace's teenage*
> *son stormed out of the room. "You*
> *try going without sleep for a whole*
> *week and see how it feels," she*
> *called after him. "I haven't had so*
> *little sleep since the year you were*
> *born!"*

Bladder difficulties. The urethral tissue is responsive to estrogen and when estrogen decreases, the urethral tissue also shrinks. This can lead to incontinence of urine. It can also lead to painful intercourse because the cervix no longer produces increased cervical mucus during sex.

Louise hadn't minded the teasing due to her occasional hot flashes, but the pain of going to the bathroom now... not to mention the embarrassment when accidents happened in public! Her incontinence had become unbearable.

Decreased libido. A woman in perimenopause can have a decrease in sexual desire. She may not want to have sex as much as she did before. Sometimes, this is not a problem as the couple becomes adjusted to the change in sexual activity and desire, however other couples may not be as lucky and this situation may lead to tension and problems in the relationship.

Janeen cringed when her husband snuck up behind her and lovingly kissed her neck. She didn't want to feel this way, but somehow romance just wasn't on her mind as much these days. She just had no desire.

Decreased ability to get pregnant. The rate of ovulation goes down during perimenopause so the woman has a reduction in the ability to get pregnant. Pregnancy can still happen, however, so if you do not want to get pregnant, you should still continue to use some form of birth control until menopause occurs.

> *When her husband rolled on top, Liza nudged him and pointed to the condom drawer. "But this is the part of this hot flash and mood swing business that I've been looking forward to," he replied. She nudged him again.*

Osteopenia. The strength of the bones depends on high circulating levels of estrogen. As estrogen levels decline, the bone mass decreases and there is a risk for osteoporosis that can increase a woman's risk of having bone fractures.

> *Janie was having back pain that just wasn't getting better. Every day, she had pain in her upper back— especially when turning to the right. She went for an x-ray that showed a fracture of her vertebra. Her doctor gave her a prescription to prevent further bone loss.*

3 | Symptoms Of Menopause

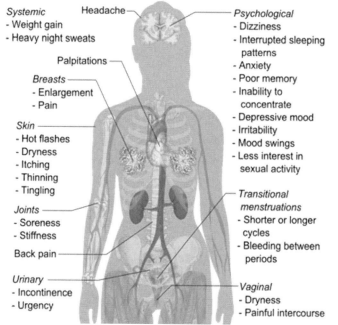

Symptoms of
Menopause

Systemic
- Weight gain
- Heavy night sweats

Headache

Psychological
- Dizziness
- Interrupted sleeping patterns
- Anxiety
- Poor memory
- Inability to concentrate
- Depressive mood
- Irritability
- Mood swings
- Less interest in sexual activity

Palpitations

Breasts
- Enlargement
- Pain

Skin
- Hot flashes
- Dryness
- Itching
- Thinning
- Tingling

Joints
- Soreness
- Stiffness

Back pain

Transitional menstruations
- Shorter or longer cycles
- Bleeding between periods

Urinary
- Incontinence
- Urgency

Vaginal
- Dryness
- Painful intercourse

As menopause approaches and the periods stop, the symptoms resulting from low estrogen levels become obvious. Common symptoms of menopause include the following:

Irregular or no more periods. The periods will begin to become irregular and will eventually stop. When you haven't had a period for 12 months in a row, it means you have reached menopause.

> *Shannon tossed the boxes of sanitary napkins and tampons into the trash can. She wasn't sure whether it was a cause to mourn or celebrate, but it had been a year since her last period.*

Increased hot flashes. The hot flashes may be similar to those in perimenopause but can be more frequent and more intense. Most hot flashes last as little as 30 seconds or as long as 10 minutes before you feel better. About 2/3 of all women will experience hot flashes as a part of their menopausal symptoms.

> *Always dressed in layers now, Petal never knew when the next hot flash was coming, or how long it might last. She just knew that her face felt like it was on fire, and then she would be drenched in embarrassing sweat.*

Vaginal dryness. Without the protective effect of estrogen and progesterone, the cervix and vagina do not secrete as much fluid. This can result in pain with intercourse as well as an increased risk of yeast infections, bladder infections, and vaginal itching. It is best treated with a water-based lubricating gel such as KY jelly.

Mandy's girlfriend was trying to be understanding. She'd brought home a variety of lubes to try, so she had to explain why the water-based ones were better choices.

Sleeping difficulties. While in menopause, sleep can be difficult. You may have difficulty getting to sleep at night or may wake earlier in the morning, with difficulty falling back to sleep. Good sleep habits can help prevent this complication.

Cassandra stared at the clock, willing the nighttime hours to pass. As she tossed and turned, she couldn't remember the last time she'd slept through the whole night.

Incontinence of Urine. Women in menopause may experience an increase in the urge to urinate, or incontinence of urine. Stress incontinence can occur, which is the kind of incontinence that occurs when coughing, lifting heavy objects, or sneezing. Urge incontinence is the type of incontinence that causes you to have sudden urges to void, sometimes not making it to the toilet before urinating.

> *Andrea no longer found the off and on incontinence funny. Allergy season had arrived, and every sneeze was the enemy.*

Bladder infections. Women in menopause may have more bladder infections than normal. This is because the lack of estrogen has resulted in atrophy of the urethral lining so that bacteria have a greater chance of traveling up to the bladder, resulting in an infection. Drinking plenty of water can help reduce the chances of getting a bladder infection.

> *Linda carried and refilled her water bottle with religious fervor. Her best friend Sandy seemed to have another bladder infection every month and there was NO WAY she wanted to suffer the same pain.*

Decreased sex drive. The lack of male and female hormones in the woman's blood can result in a decreased interest in sex. There may be fewer orgasms or no orgasms at all. This can be treated with prescription medications that help a woman achieve an orgasm.

> *It was bad enough for Nancy that she no longer craved the physical intimacy she'd once enjoyed with her lover. Now even when the magic moments arrived, no matter what they tried, she couldn't even come close to orgasm.*

Vaginal dryness. The walls of the vagina become thinner because they no longer have estrogen to build up the lining. This can cause pain on intercourse that can be managed with over-the-counter vaginal lubricants. Estrogen in a vaginal ring can restore some of the vaginal dryness.

> *Sally was almost at her wits end. She didn't want to give up the lovemaking she and her partner had shared for decades, but now it hurt so much she shied away every time the opportunity presented itself.*

Mood swings. Mood swings and depressive symptoms can result from a lack of estrogen. The fluctuations in female hormones affect the brain as well as the rest of the body so that there are reductions in the neurotransmitters necessary to maintain a healthy mood.

> *Vickie didn't even find the mood swing jokes funny anymore. Why did every conversation have to come back to her menopause symptoms? It was as bad as the period questions she got when she was younger.*

Skin and Hair Changes. Menopause can increase the rate of hair loss so that the hair will be thinner than before menopause. There will be a loss of body fat and collagen so that the skin will become more wrinkled, and will have decreased elasticity and increased dryness.

> *Jan stared mournfully into the mirror. Her thinning hair had been bad enough, but now the age lines around her eyes made her look and feel decades older. What to do?*

Menopausal symptoms can last a few months or a few years. They can also last for a few weeks and then go away for many months before starting up again. Most women will have decreased

menopausal symptoms once they finally go through the menopausal stage.

Hot Flashes

Hot flashes are perhaps the most common symptom of menopause. Statistically 3/4 of all menopausal women experience hot flashes[2] and it's usually the most uncomfortable symptom. Hot flashes can go on for several years before stopping and can be treated in a couple of ways.

Some women choose to replace the estrogen and progesterone the ovaries are no longer making.

Estrogen replacement therapy or HRT is a prescription treatment for hot flashes.

Estrogen is given by patch, vaginal ring, or pill and progesterone can be given by pill. They are usually given together in order to prevent a buildup of the uterine lining that occurs when a woman takes unopposed estrogen.

---

[2] Woods NF, Mitchell ES. Symptoms during the perimenopause: prevalence, severity, trajectory, and significance in women's lives. *Am J Med*. 2005;118 (suppl 12B):14-24.

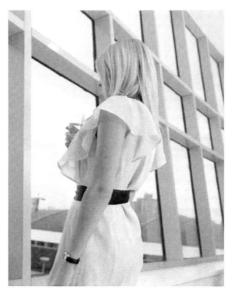

Progesterone will help decrease the thickness of the uterine lining so that there are either regular periods (when the hormones are taken cyclically) or vaginal spotting if the hormones are taken every day. Women with a uterus must have progesterone when taking estrogen.

Other women use lifestyle changes or natural remedies for the management of hot flashes. These include the following:

- Stay away from warm areas and do not sleep with warm blankets or warm pajamas.
- Avoid hot foods and drinks that can heat up the body and trigger hot flashes.

- Decrease alcohol intake as this can increase the amount of facial flushing you get with hot flashes.
- Decrease the amount of stress you are under.
- Quit smoking or do not start smoking during this time of your life.
- Wear several layers of clothing that can be peeled off when you begin to get hot.
- Buy a portable fan so you can fan yourself when you get hot.
- Exercise regularly every day for at least thirty minutes. Try not to exercise right before you sleep as this can affect your ability to fall asleep.
- Decrease stress through the use of biofeedback, meditation, yoga, qi gong, or Tai chi. These are natural ways of reducing the amount of perceived stress.
- Try this breathing technique when you get a hot flash: take in deep abdominal breaths, in through your nose and out through the mouth. Breathe slowly, only 5-7 times per minute.
- Use a bedside fan to remain cool at night.
- Drink cool water if you wake up with a hot flash or night sweats during your sleep.

- Use a cooling pillow or turn your pillow often so that you don't have to sleep on the hot side of the pillow all night. Keep a cool pack under the pillow so you can flip to a cool pillow during the night.
- Try to lose weight if you are overweight. Women who are obese have more problems with hot flashes than women of normal weight. You can lose weight through healthy eating and maintaining an exercise program that will help decrease your hot flashes.
- Acupuncture. A trained acupuncturist can help you reduce the blocked flow of qi energy so as to decrease the number and intensity of hot flashes.
- Try eating soy or taking soy supplements. You can get more soy, which contains isoflavones that mimic estrogen, by eating things like soymilk, tempeh, tofu, or roasted soy nuts. One soy supplement is called Promensil, which can be purchased over the counter, but ask your doctor first.
- Try herbal remedies such as black cohosh. This is an herb that has been found to decrease the incidence of hot flashes in some studies.

One study showed that exercise decreased the incidence and intensity of hot flashes[3]. The study was done on 21 women who were having menopausal symptoms. Fourteen of the women took part in an exercise program for four months, while the rest did not change their exercise activities. After the study, the women completed a questionnaire that asked them about how many hot flashes they had and how intense the hot flashes were. They also cause hot flashes by placing the participants in a hot water suit and recorded their body responses.

The exercising participants took part in a gym-based exercise program, in which they used a stationary bicycle, a treadmill, a cross trainer and/or a rowing machine. They were asked to exercise initially for thirty minutes, later increasing to 45-minute exercise sessions a day for at least five days a week.

After the 16-week study, the researchers measured the incidence and severity of the hot flashes each woman experienced. They found that, in the women who exercised, the amount of sweating during a hot flash was markedly reduced. There was a decrease in blood flow to the forearms by 7 percent and a

---

[3] Bailey, TG, Cable, NT, Aziz, N, Atkinson, G, Cuthbertson, DG, Low, DA, Jones, H. Exercise training reduces the acute physiological severity of post-menopausal hot flushes. J. Physiology 2015 https://doi.org/10.1113/JP271456

decrease in blood flow to the chest by 9 percent. There was also a decrease in blood flow to the brain in those women who exercised.

Women who did not exercise had no difference in the incidence and severity of hot flashes. While the study was small, it did indicate the possibility that exercise could help women with hot flashes.

Jennifer started having hot flashes in her early 50s. She wasn't sure what was going on. She was just feeling "weird most of the time." In addition to hot flashes, she started craving sweets when she never had before. She also started craving coffee. Her hot flashes were so debilitating that they woke her 2-3 times per night. She had hot flashes every 5-15 minutes! One time she was in a staff meeting and suddenly became hot and sweaty. Her face was so red like a beet! The men she was working with laughed at her, but her manager (a woman) understood. Thankfully, she wasn't with a group of strangers.

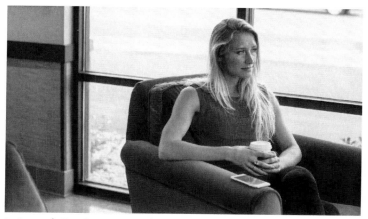

Mood Swings and Depression

Women approaching or in menopause are subject to mood swings and increased irritability. Typically, this occurs as a result of hormone fluctuations.

Some menopausal women also suffer from depression. The reasons for this are not completely clear but the hypothesis is that the lack of estrogen affects the amount of brain neurotransmitters responsible for prevention of depression. When neurotransmitters like serotonin and norepinephrine are decreased, the risk for depression increases.

Women in menopause may need to take prescription antidepressants in order to control depressive symptoms. These include many of the SSRI (selective serotonin reuptake inhibitors) antidepressants, which increase the levels of serotonin in the brain and decrease depressive symptoms.

Some of these include Lexapro, Prozac, Paxil, Celexa, and Wellbutrin. Technically, Wellbutrin is a SNRI antidepressant, which means it increases both serotonin and norepinephrine in the brain.

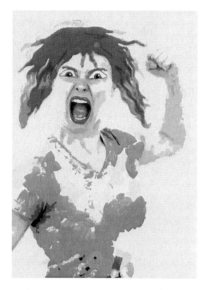

Some women have more anxiety than depression in menopause. Doctors can prescribe short courses of anti-anxiety medications to relieve these uncomfortable symptoms. Anti-anxiety medications include Xanax, Klonopin, and Ativan.

There are numerous natural remedies for mood swings:

- Make sure you eat a diet of healthy foods. Avoid processed foods and foods containing sugar, excessive salt, and high fructose corn syrup.
- Eat smaller portions. If you get food cravings, try eating a small snack instead of loading up on unhealthy foods.
- Take in at least five portions of vegetables per day and at least 2 servings of fruit per day. Eat foods that are high in color as these contain healthful phytonutrients that can improve your mood and cognitive function.
- Eat organic foods whenever they are available. Try to avoid foods that may contain hormones, pesticides, herbicides, and food preservatives.
- When eating fruits, stick to whole fruits instead of the juice of the fruit. Whole fruits contain fiber, which are good for your bowels.
- Decrease your intake of caffeine. This means consuming less caffeine-containing sodas, black tea, and coffee.
- Instead of black tea, switch to healthier green tea or purified water to decrease caffeine intake.

- Eat berries for a healthy treat. They contain healthful antioxidants, which scavenge for oxygen free radicals and can improve the way your brain works.
- Eat healthy fats like olive oil, coconut oil, avocados, and natural fats. Remember that nature doesn't make bad fats.
- Eat foods that are high in vitamin C, including citrus fruits, red peppers, and spinach. These contain antioxidants that can decrease the dryness of your skin and can decrease wrinkling.
- Increase the amount of omega 3 fatty acids in your diet. You can find omega 3 fatty acids by eating higher amounts of flaxseed oil, walnuts, and fatty fish.
- Eat foods high in antioxidant and anti-inflammatory capabilities. You can increase the anti-inflammatory effect by adding turmeric, cayenne pepper, garlic, and rosemary to the foods you eat.
- Get more exercise. You can do this by increasing the amount of walking you do, by cycling, swimming, or engaging in any exercise that gets your heart rate going and increases your respiratory rate.

- Stop smoking. Women who smoke often have worse menopausal symptoms when compared to women who do not smoke and will, on average, start menopausal symptoms 2 years earlier than those who don't smoke.
- Avoid perfumes as these can disrupt the balance of chemicals in your body.
- Engage in stress-relieving activities. This can be enjoying a hobby or taking the time to read a book.
- De-clutter your life so you have fewer things to be stressed about.
- Try meditation, massage therapy, qi gong, yoga, or tai chi to reduce the perception of stress in your life.
- Try herbal therapy. A practitioner in Traditional Chinese Medicine is trained in the herbs that can reduce menopausal symptoms and can guide you to the right herbs to take, such as black cohosh.
- Try taking bioidentical hormones. These are estrogen and progesterone and sometimes testosterone depending on your doctor. They are usually rubbed into the skin, and are identical in chemistry to the actual hormones you'll find in your body. Some practitioners

say that these are safer to take than chemically manufactured hormones.

- Support your adrenal glands by taking vitamins that support the glands. Your adrenal glands also make some reproductive hormones so, if they are supported, you may have fewer symptoms of hot flashes, and night sweats.

- Linda just didn't understand what was going on. One minute she was nice to her husband, the next she was biting his head off. She started paying attention to her self-talk and journaling more. With these tools, she was able to talk herself down more often than not, until that time she ended up on a bridge after a 50-mile drive. She took a wrong turn mere feet from her destination and added 30 minutes to the trip. That warranted a scream.

Fatigue

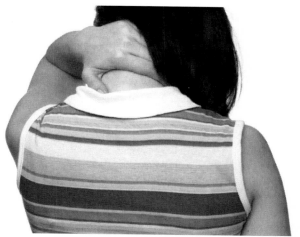

Menopause is a time when many women feel run down and fatigued. Part of the problem is the increased perception of stress and another part is the decrease in restful sleep that comes with menopause.

Stress reduction techniques can reduce the fatigue seen in menopause. Exercises like guided imagery, meditation, qi gong, and tai chi can also reduce stress so you have more energy as well as increased mental clarity.

Fatigue can be managed by developing better sleep habits. This will help you go to sleep when you are tired and can keep you sleeping longer. Some good sleep habits include:

- Use your bedroom for sleep and sex only. Do not use your bed for watching television.
- Sleep in a dark and quiet environment. Use dark shades if it is still light out when you go to bed.
- Use a white noise machine or a fan if there is a lot of ambient noise. This can soothe your nerves and help you fall asleep more easily.
- Exercise about five hours before going to sleep. Do not exercise right before bedtime as this can be activating and interfere with falling asleep.
- Do not eat a big meal before bedtime. Eat at least 3 hours before falling asleep so your body has a chance to digest the food before bedtime.
- Do not smoke before sleeping, as this can be overly stimulating.
- Do not drink alcohol just before sleep. While alcohol is technically a depressant, it will not help you fall asleep.

Don't be afraid to take naps during the day. A nap of even twenty minutes can fight fatigue and can get you through the rest of the day. Set an alarm if you are afraid you might nap for too long, as this can make it hard to fall asleep at night.

If fatigue is a problem and sleep is difficult, talk to your doctor about a short course of a medication that can help you sleep. There are several sleep preparations that can be prescribed, some of which are not addictive.

- Nora slumped at her desk. For as long as she could remember she was exhausted. She couldn't sleep. It's such a viscous cycle, she thought. I go to bed exhausted, I toss and turn, and then I have to get up and go to work in the morning. When will this end?

Stress

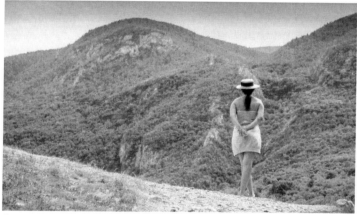

Stress can increase the frequency and intensity of hot flashes. Anything you can do to reduce your level of stress will help you feel better during this time of your life. If the stress has reached a level where you are anxious, your doctor can prescribe anti-anxiety medications that will reduce your perception of stress. Some of these anxiolytic agents include Valium, clonazepam, Ativan, and Xanax.

There are natural ways of reducing stress:

- Aerobic exercises like running, jogging, walking, swimming, and cycling can reduce stress. Exercise should ideally be done for thirty minutes a day on most days of the week.
- Anaerobic exercise, such as weight machines and lifting weights, can be done about twice a week to increase muscle tone and lessen stress.
- Meditation or guided imagery can help with stress. In meditation, you focus on breathing and on progressively relaxing your muscles to induce a completely relaxed but aware state. This can be done sitting up in a comfortable position or lying down on your bed or on a mat. In guided imagery, focus on your breath and imagine yourself in a peaceful location, focusing on the sights, sounds, and smells of being in that location. You can take yourself there whenever you feel you are under stress in order to reduce your perception of stress.

Apps like Headspace and Omvana have many excellent guided meditations.

- Yoga, tai chi, and QiGong are wonderful mind-body exercises to relieve stress.
- Massage, a spa day, or even a weekend in nature can do wonders to reduce stress levels.
- Some people get rid of their stress by de-stressing their lives. To do this, tackle those things that negatively affect the stress in your life. This might mean quitting a stressful job, managing a stressful relationship, or handling stressful finances.
- Take up a hobby that reduces the impact of stress on your life.
- Make yourself a priority; make sure to intentionally relax several times per day.

Phyllis and her husband were having one of "those" discussions again. Their son wanted to stay out late, and they had differing opinions on what was acceptable. Before menopause, she would have talked to her husband about it without difficulty. Now, she just didn't have the patience. It seemed he was being irrational and not using common sense.

Vaginal Dryness

The decrease in estrogen produced by the ovaries can lead to vaginal dryness. This can result in vaginal and vulvar itching, as well as pain during intercourse. Fortunately, there are things you can do to reduce the symptoms of vaginal dryness in menopause.

First, discontinue using harsh soap on the inner lips of the vagina. Instead, just use plain water to clean these parts of your genitals. Use white toilet paper that has no scent in it and wash your underwear in soaps that contain no perfumes or dyes.

Don't use any anti-cling sheets or fabric softeners when you do laundry, as these can be irritating. Don't use perfumed douches or lotions on the inner lips of the vulva.

There are many lubricants you can purchase over the counter in order to maintain vaginal lubrication. Some of these include the following:

- KY™ jelly
- FemGlide™
- Just Like Me™
- Astroglide™
- Pre-Seed™
- Summer's Eve Lubricant™
- Slippery Stuff™

- Pure Pleasure™
- ID Millennium™

Avoid using petroleum-based lubricants such as petroleum jelly as they do not actually lubricate the vagina and can actually increase the irritation. They can also cause latex condoms to break.

Prescription (from a doctor) estrogen-based vaginal products include the following:

- Estrace vaginal cream
- Vagifem vaginal tablet
- Neo-Estrone cream
- Premarin Cream
- Estring vaginal ring

Any of these vaginal moisturizers can effectively reduce the vaginal dryness and can make intercourse more pleasurable. Try the over-the-counter preparations first and, if these don't work, go to the prescription products.

The vaginal estrogen creams and tablets are safer than taking oral estrogen because they deliver estrogen directly to the vaginal tissues and are not absorbed appreciably by the rest of the body. They can thicken the vaginal mucosa and can increase lubrication.

Warming Lubricants

You can also use "warming" vaginal lubricants. These are available over the counter and are designed to increase sexual responsiveness by containing a small amount of capsaicin in the lubricant.

These types of lubricants can be very helpful in increasing sexual responsiveness but some women say the lubricants increase irritation of the vaginal tissues.

Vaginal Moisturizers

Vaginal moisturizers can be applied on a regular basis to moisturize the vaginal tissue and have effectiveness that lasts about 3-4 days. They work by mimicking the vagina's normal vaginal secretions.

They are usually applied using an applicator and are available over the counter or online. You can use both vaginal moisturizers and vaginal lubricants together to reduce vaginal dryness.

Some women prefer using vaginal estrogen treatments. These involve the use of the products listed above. Estrogen vaginal treatments are known to increase the blood flow to the vagina so that the vagina has increased elasticity and thickness.

These products offer lasting relief of vaginal dryness and can be used on a long-term basis. They are available by prescription and take a while to take effect.

Oral Estrogen Therapy

If you need more relief of menopausal symptoms than just vaginal dryness, you may want to use oral estrogen therapy. This can help all of the symptoms of menopause, including hot flashes, night sweats, mood swings, urinary tract symptoms, and vaginal dryness.

For severe vaginal atrophy, however, the prescription vaginal creams, rings, or tablets are what are primarily recommended.

Local vaginal estrogen therapy is very effective, with about 93 percent of women indicating significant improvement in their symptoms.[4,5,6,7]

Up to 75% of women indicate that the pain on intercourse resolves using this type of therapy. Always use the lowest effective dose and talk to your doctor if you have a history of breast cancer as estrogen therapy may be contraindicated in women who have had breast cancer.

How To Use Estrogen Vaginal Preparations
If you are using estrogen-containing vaginal cream, apply small amounts in the range of 0.5 to 1.0 grams in an applicator 2-3 times per week. Do not use prior to intercourse as the estrogen in the cream can be

---

[4] Barentsen R, van de Weijer PH, Schram JH. Continuous low dose estradiol released from a vaginal ring versus estriol vaginal cream for urogenital atrophy. *Eur J Obstet Gynecol Reprod Biol* 1997;71:73-80.

[5] Simunic V, Banovic I, Ciglar S, et al. Local estrogen treatment in patients with urogenital symptoms. *Int J Gynaecol Obstet* 2003;82:187-197.

[6]Eriksen PS, Rasmussen H. Low-dose 17 beta-estradiol vaginal tablets in the treatment of atrophic vaginitis: a double-blind placebo controlled study. Eur J Obstet Gynecol Reprod Biol 1992;44:137-144.

[7] Lose G, Englev E. Oestradiol-releasing vaginal ring versus oestriol vaginal pessaries in the treatment of bothersome lower urinary tract symptoms. *Br J Obstet Gynaecol*2000;107:1029-1034.

absorbed in the man's skin and possibly cause adverse effects.

If you are using the Estring vaginal ring, insert it into the vagina, where it is worn for three months before replacement. It resides near the cervix and does not have to be removed prior to having intercourse. Estring is used exclusively for vaginal dryness and is different from Femring, which is a type of vaginal estrogen-containing ring that has a higher dose of estrogen for the management of menopause symptoms.

When using the vaginal tablet known as Vagifem, simply use your finger or an applicator to insert the tablet about twice weekly. Vaginal tablets are generally less messy than the estrogen-containing creams.

The type of vaginal estrogen-containing product you use depends on your and your doctor's preferences. Individual responses vary, so you may need to experiment with products if one does not provide the desired results. You can use lubricants and moisturizers in addition to estrogen-containing vaginal products, as they do not generally have adverse affects. As always, double check with your doctor or pharmacist before adding an over-the-counter product to a prescription one.

Jennifer loves her husband but doesn't want to get pregnant. When she tried to have sex with her husband, she couldn't because the condoms just hurt. She knows her husband loves her, but she just doesn't want to have a child. Her solution was to stop having sex. She knows it's a big problem for him. This has become a source of stress in the marriage. Like many people, she's embarrassed about sex and doesn't always want to have oral sex. Anal is OUT of the question. So she doesn't want to go to bed and doesn't sleep well.

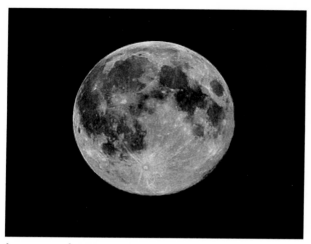

Insomnia

Almost 50% of perimenopausal and menopausal women will suffer from insomnia. [8] Insomnia is defined as not being able to get to sleep once you have gone to bed, or getting up earlier than you would like to once you have achieved sleep.

Many women develop symptoms of menopause-related insomnia in their late 30s to early 40s.

[8] Baker FC, Wolfson AR, Lee KA. Association of sociodemographic, lifestyle, and health factors with sleep quality and daytime sleepiness in women: findings from the 2007 National Sleep Foundation "Sleep in America Poll." *J Womens Health (Larchmt)* 2009;18:841-849.

Some Of The Causes Of This Include The Following:

- **Changes in Hormones.** During the perimenopausal and menopausal years, the ovaries decrease their production of estrogen and progesterone, which are responsible for inducing sleep. A shift in the ratio of estrogen to progesterone can cause you to have difficulty falling asleep.

- **Hot flashes.** Hot flashes induce a sensation of heat and sweating that can wake you. It is caused by an upsurge of adrenaline, which interferes with the sleep process.

- **Mood swings.** Menopause can trigger depressive episodes in up to twenty percent of women. [9] Life stressors can add to the difficulty in sleeping. The mood swings are a result of a change in neurotransmitters in the brain that are helpful in helping you get to sleep.

---

[9] Soares CN. New York, Arlington, VA: American Psychiatric Publishing; 2004. Perimenopause-related Mood Disturbance: An Update on Risk Factors and Novel Treatment Strategies Available. In: Meeting Program and Abstracts. Psychopharmacology and Reproductive Transitions Symposium. American Psychiatric Association 157th Annual Meeting; May 1.6, 2004; pp. 51–61.

- **Social issues.** Menopause is a time of life changes that can interfere with sleep. It can be a time of relationship difficulties, difficulties with your children, and other midlife crises that make it difficult to relax enough to sleep.

If you are finding it difficult to sleep because of perimenopausal or menopausal symptoms, see your healthcare provider for help.

To improve sleep, adhere to a predictable bedtime routine and establish good sleep habits. Hormone replacement may help as well. Discuss hormone replacement with your health care practitioner.

If, after trying the steps above, you are still suffering from sleep deprivation or insomnia, discuss with your doctor. He or she may want to prescribe hormone therapy or sleep aids.

Practice the sleep habits discussed above. Keep your room as cool as possible in order to combat hot flashes and make every attempt to go to sleep at the same time each night and wake up at the same time every morning. Keep a cold rag by your bedside so you can cool down after waking from a hot flash or night sweat.

Hormone replacement therapy can help control the hot flashes and may help you stay asleep at night. This type of therapy should be short-term as there is some research evidence (the Women's Health Initiative) that indicates that hormone replacement therapy is a risk factor for heart disease. For those women in perimenopause, low-dose birth control pills can be used instead of hormone replacement therapy. The current U.S. Food and Drug Administration recommendation for menopausal hormone therapy is that it should be used at the lowest dose for the shortest period of time to reach treatment goals.

The following herbal remedies may improve sleep: valerian root, kava, chamomile and St. John's wort. A calming chamomile tea can be relaxing if consumed just before sleep. The others can be taken as a supplement purchased over the counter at a pharmacy or health food store. Make sure your healthcare provider knows you are taking these medications and discuss drug interactions with a pharmacist or your doctor before starting a new supplement.

If all else fails, consider prescription therapy. Besides benzodiazepine therapy, specific for sleep, you can try non-addictive forms of sleep aids such as trazodone, Vistaril, and melatonin (over the counter in the U.S. and prescription in Europe).

Natural forms of sleep induction include acupuncture, acupressure, or shiatsu massage. These are based on the idea that qi energy in the body is being blocked, interfering with sleep.

Yoga may help you get a good night's sleep. Other things that may help with sleep include relaxation therapy and exercise (at least 5 hours before bedtime) earlier in the day before you go to bed.

Misty rolled over, again. When she went to bed it had taken her over 30 minutes to fall asleep because her brain wouldn't shut off. Now, 3 hours later, she awoke in a pool of sweat, feeling like she was on fire. She got up and went to the bathroom (a nightly occurrence), but was freezing by the time she returned to bed to attempt to get back to sleep... lying on the wet sheets. She resolved to try chamomile tea before bed tomorrow, if she could remember.

Weight Gain

There is a natural tendency to gain weight as a result of menopause for reasons that are not completely clear. It may have something to do with changes in metabolism around the time of menopause. There are, however, things you can do to prevent or address weight gain associated with menopause.

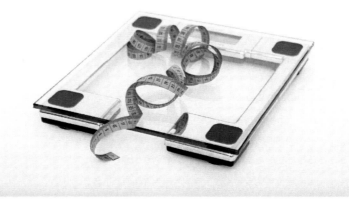

Increasing physical activity should improve your metabolism and stave off menopausal weight gain. Engage in some form of aerobic activity at least 30 minutes a day 4-5 days per week. Aerobic activity can be any form of exercise that increases the heart rate and respiratory rate. Common forms of aerobic exercise include brisk walking, jogging, swimming, and bicycling. Other women engage in exercises associated with hobbies, such as gardening, tennis, or golf.

Perform anaerobic exercise on the days of the week you don't do aerobic exercise. Anaerobic exercise involves lifting weights or using weight machines at a local gym. Anaerobic exercise does burn some calories but it is really effective in increasing muscle tone and improving muscle mass. Muscle tissue has a higher metabolic rate than other tissues of the body, so increasing your muscle mass will result in a higher caloric burn (resting metabolic rate).

Menopause is a great time to learn about healthy eating and apply that learning to your daily habits. Eat a diet that is moderately low in calories and that contains plenty of vegetables, fish, and lean meats with a moderate amount of fruit. You do not necessarily have to count calories unless you are trying to lose weight.

Reduce your intake of processed foods, fried foods, fast foods, and vegetable oils (like canola, safflower, etc.). These are not healthy and can contribute not only to weight gain but also to an increase in inflammation, cardiovascular disease and diabetes. If you are already diabetic, you should take on a 2000-calorie a day diabetic (low-carb, no added sugar) diet that ensures your blood sugars stay stable and will help you lose weight.

It is better to prevent weight gain than it is to take the weight off once it has already been gained. The earlier in your life that you adopt healthy practices of eating and exercising often, the less problem you will have with weight gain associated with menopause.

You should aim to have a body mass index (BMI) of 25 or less. You can calculate your BMI online using an online BMI calculator or chart.

- A BMI of 25 or less is normal.
- A BMI of more than 25 but less than 30 means you are overweight.
- A BMI of between 30 and 40 means that you are obese.
- If your BMI is greater than 40, you are considered to be morbidly obese.
- BMI is not accurate for very muscular individuals.
    - Faith looked in the mirror. Her belly was expanding around the middle and she didn't understand why. No matter what she tried, she just couldn't shift the weight. She thought to herself, "I'm having incessant hot flashes where I feel like my face is on fire every 20 minutes, my mood is all over the place, and now I look like I'm 9-months pregnant! What am I going to do?" She knew she hadn't changed her eating habits. She was eating all the same foods she had eaten before. She started

feeling less and less like herself and more and more like an alien had taken control of her body.

Memory Loss And Brain Fog

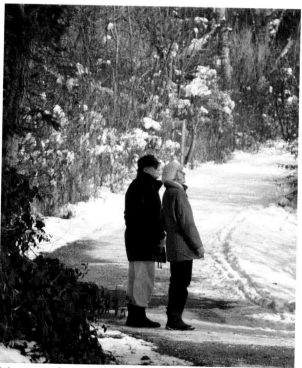

Memory loss is one of the more common symptoms of perimenopause and menopause. In fact, about

60% of women experiencing perimenopause and menopause have some symptoms of memory loss.[10]

In laymen's terms, memory loss in menopause is called "brain fog" and it involves feeling as though you can't remember things as well as you used to and are walking around with a muddled head.

The type of memory loss seen during perimenopause and menopause usually involves forgetting newly acquired verbal information and having difficulty with concentration.

Typical brain fog symptoms include forgetting people's names (particularly new names of people you just met), forgetting tasks in the middle of trying to do them, or forgetting where you left things, such as your car keys.

Fortunately, the problem is not permanent and does not mean you are becoming demented. In fact, research out of the University of California, Los Angeles, from 2009 tracked more than 2,000 menopausal women regarding their memory loss. The study found that women's symptoms of learning

---

[10] Maturitas. 2015 Nov;82(3):288-90. doi: 10.1016/j.maturitas.2015.07.023. Epub 2015 Aug 11.

disability and memory loss returned to normal after menopause.[11]

Why Does Brain Fog Occur?

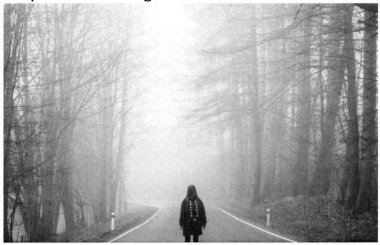

Hormone fluctuations are usually at fault, just like the other symptoms of menopause. When the levels of estrogen fluctuate during the perimenopausal state, women can get various symptoms, including hot flashes, night sweats, decreased mood, vaginal dryness, urinary tract problems, and mood swings.

In addition, women in menopause often do not sleep well. These sleep difficulties are also caused by fluctuations in estrogen levels and contribute to the

---

[11] Greendale GA, Huang MH, Wight RG, et al. Effects of the menopause transition and hormone use on cognitive performance in midlife women. Neurology. 2009;72(21):1850–1857.

inability to concentrate and the memory difficulties associated with brain fog.

Estrogen is required by a woman to sleep well, pay attention to things, have good short-term memory, acquire language skills, and keep your mood stable.

The presence of hot flashes in menopause seems to be related to a loss of memory, particularly verbal memory, which involves remembering words. A study out of the University of Illinois, Chicago, in 2008 revealed that moderate to severe hot flashes are an indicator of memory loss.[12]

The study looked at 29 menopausal and perimenopausal women, who had at least moderate to severe vasomotor symptoms (hot flashes). Those women who reported more hot flashes did more poorly on verbal memory testing.

Treating Brain Fog

- **Try hormone replacement therapy.** While hormone replacement therapy (HRT) is usually given for the treatment of hot flashes, it can also improve memory and concentration. A study out of UCLA showed

---

[12] Maki PM, Drogos LL, Rubin LH, Banuvar S, Shulman LP, Geller SE. Objective hot flashes are negatively related to verbal memory performance in midlife women. *Menopause*. 2008;15(5):848-56.

that giving HRT to perimenopausal women had a positive impact on memory. Remember that HRT is not without risk, and can increase the risk of female-related cancers and heart disease, especially when given after age 60. If you are considering HRT, discuss the pros and cons with your physician to assess the risks and benefits of using this type of therapy.

- **Get plenty of sleep.** Sleep disturbances are extremely common in menopause. If you can turn that around and get more sleep, you can improve your memory and other brain fog symptoms. In order to sleep better, you may need to practice better sleep habits. This means developing a sleep ritual, such as limiting alcohol and caffeine before sleeping, turning off screens 30 minutes before bed, keeping the room cool and free of distractions, or relaxing in a warm bath before going to bed.

- **Eat a healthy diet.** Eating better can improve your memory. Foods that contain omega-3 fatty acids (such as is found in cold water, fatty fish) seem to help memory loss caused by menopause. A review study out of UCLA indicated that omega-3 fatty acids could be beneficial in controlling the memory loss and improving memory.[13] You can also get these types of fatty acids from kiwi and walnuts. Folate is a water-soluble vitamin B that helps your brain improve its ability to remember. Folate can be found in the diet by eating plenty of leafy green vegetables or by taking a folate supplement.

- **Little to no alcohol.** No wine, or less than 2 glasses per week. Red wine may be better than other forms of alcohol due to its high concentration of resveratrol. Resveratrol scavenges for free radicals in the brain. It is unclear if there is truly a benefit to drinking red wine. No alcohol is the best amount of alcohol for humans. To decrease inflammation eat foods high in turmeric (e.g., curry) or taken as a supplement. Turmeric is also high in antioxidants that may help improve brain fog symptoms.

- **Ginkgo Biloba.** While many believe that gingko biloba enhances brain function, it hasn't held up to that claim in the U.S. Research in Germany, however, has indicated its usefulness for memory loss. It is commonly

[13] Gómez-Pinilla, Fernando Brain foods: the effects of nutrients on brain function. Nature Reviews Neuroscience. 2008/07/01/online. Nature Publishing Group.

used in Germany to improve memory and decrease the onset of dementia. Have a discussion with your doctor before taking this herb, as there can be some drug-to-herb interactions, depending on what medications you are taking.

- **Develop your memory.** If you feel as though brain fog is a problem, try using memory tips to make sure you don't forget everything. Write things down, break complex tasks into separate steps, and play games like Sudoku, Scrabble, and crossword puzzles.

- **Decrease stress.** Menopause can be a time when stressful life events are more likely to occur. You may have to take care of teenage children, balance responsibilities at home and work, or be the caregiver for your elderly parent. If you cannot change these things in your life, try stress-reducing techniques like meditation, yoga, and tai chi to decrease the perception of stress and improve your memory.

Brain fog symptoms don't affect all women in menopause but if you are experiencing these symptoms, there are things you can do to combat the problem.

Even if you do nothing, your memory loss symptoms and other brain function activities will likely return to baseline levels when menopause ends.

Tabitha said, "Hey Harry! How's it going?" She and Harry had worked together for several months. They saw each other in meetings, in the kitchen, and around the water cooler. He always answered her when she called him Harry. One day, he said to her, "Tabitha, can I ask you a serious question?" She said, "Sure, go ahead." He said, "Why do you keep calling me Harry?" She answered, "That's your name, isn't it?" He replied, "No, actually it's Gary and it has been since birth!" They laughed it off, but Tabitha started wondering about her memory.

4 | Hormonal Changes In Menopause

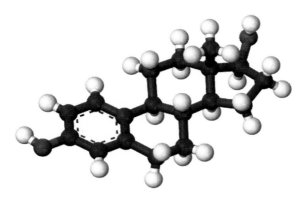

As perimenopause turns to menopause, the amount of estrogen and progesterone produced by the ovaries declines to low levels. This has a major impact on the body. The protective effect of estrogen against heart disease goes away so that a postmenopausal woman has an increased risk of developing heart disease, including heart attacks, stroke, and peripheral vascular disease.

Bone Density

If a woman does not take extra calcium or has early menopause, she is at a much higher risk of developing thinning of the bones, known as osteoporosis.

This can lead to bony fractures of the back, wrist, and hip. It often takes very little injury (or no injury at all) to cause these bones to fracture, particularly the vertebra. Fortunately, bone density can be checked and there are medications available that will keep the bones strong.

Andi unloaded the dishwasher slower now. The pain in her wrist still reminded her of how easily it had fractured when she accidentally cracked it on the door of an overhead cabinet.

Loss Of Libido

Women need their hormones to have some type of sexual arousal. Without the estrogen, progesterone, and testosterone produced by the ovaries, libido suffers. You may not feel like having sex in the same way that you did when you were younger.

Sometimes estrogen replacement therapy helps increase libido. In some cases, the woman needs to take small amounts of testosterone in order to bring the libido to normal. Talk to your healthcare provider if you think you might benefit from testosterone therapy.

The lack of estrogen affects the skin and connective tissue. The skin may become drier and need more moisturizer. The amount of collagen and elastin produced by the body decrease. This makes the skin have more wrinkles and reduced elasticity. There are many beauty products out there that can increase the collagen levels in the skin. Bone broth is another excellent way to add more collagen to your diet and skin.

The lack of estrogen also affects the health of the vaginal tissue. The vaginal lining becomes thinner or atrophies, resulting in very little lubrication. This can cause pain during intercourse and can result in thinning of the urethral tissue possibly increasing the risk of bladder infections.

How is this treated?

The use of estrogen-based vaginal creams (and other products) can improve the moisturization of the vaginal tissue. Oral estrogen replacement therapy can decrease the risk of osteoporosis but is not protective against heart disease.

SSRI (e.g., Fluoxetine or Prozac) therapy can be used for mood swings and for sleep deprivation. Other medications, such as mood stabilizers can be used to improve the overall state of your mood and emotions. There are medications available to help with sleep and herbal remedies that can help with sleep problems in menopause.

Julia and her husband both loved the results since her doctor prescribed a mild testosterone supplement. Some days it was almost like being teenagers again, and others her desire outstripped his.

5 | Hormone Replacement Therapy

In the 1990s, it was a common practice to give a woman estrogen and progesterone in order to treat hot flashes and other symptoms of menopause. This was until the Women's Health Initiative[14] indicated a risk for developing heart disease in women who took hormone replacement.

The practice of prescribing hormone replacement therapy declined after those findings. However, it is still being used today in select cases where menopausal symptoms are severe and the woman recognizes the possible risk of taking the medication. Hormone therapy is a good choice for certain women, depending on their other risk factors.

---

[14] https://www.whi.org/

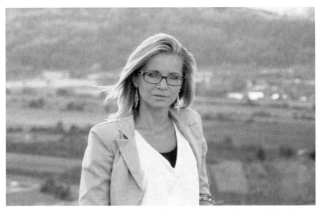

Hormone replacement therapy is also called estrogen replacement therapy, menopausal hormone therapy, or simply HRT. It is the practice of giving estrogen and progesterone (if the woman has a uterus) for the relief of the most common symptoms of menopause and for some, to slow the progress of aging.

Healthcare providers can prescribe hormone replacement therapy (HRT) while a woman is experiencing the symptoms of menopause or after menopause has already occurred.

The main purpose of hormone replacement therapy is to treat the symptoms of menopause, including thinning of bones, vaginal dryness, hot flashes, and night sweats.

By giving hormone replacement therapy, the doctor is trying to replace the hormones no longer made by the ovaries.

Estrogen is important for the body. Besides being responsible for the menstrual cycle and uterine wall thickness, it has an effect on the strength of bones, affects how the body makes use of calcium, and increases the amount of HDL ("good") cholesterol in the body.

Progesterone also plays a role in the female reproductive system. It causes the uterine lining to mature and shed at the end of the menstrual cycle.

If a woman with a uterus takes estrogen alone without progesterone for the management of menopausal symptoms, the risk of endometrial cancer (cancer of the uterus) increases. Progesterone thins the lining of the uterus so that the cells don't proliferate and cause cancerous cells to develop.

Types Of HRT

There are many ways to administer hormone replacement therapy. Talk your doctor about what kind of therapy is best for you. Here are some choices:

- **Estrogen alone.** If a woman has no uterus, she has no chance of developing uterine cancer so estrogen can be given alone as a form of hormone replacement therapy. Estrogen can be given in several ways, including a pill you take once daily, a patch you wear for a week at a time, a vaginal ring, a gel you put on your skin, or an estrogen-containing spray. Estrogen alone will control the symptoms of perimenopause and menopause but may increase the risk of developing breast cancer in women who have estrogen-sensitive breast cancer.

- **Estrogen and progesterone therapy.** This is often referred to as combination therapy. It involves giving both estrogen and a synthetic progesterone, called progestin. The progestin does not do much to reduce the hot flashes alone but is designed for women who still have their uterus in order to prevent uterine cancer.

- **Bioidentical hormone therapy.** There are compounding pharmacies that make bioidentical hormones given alone or in combination for menopausal symptoms. Bioidentical hormones are the same as the hormones in the body and must be given as a cream or gel applied to the skin where it is rapidly absorbed.

Risks Of HRT

As mentioned, there are risks to taking hormone replacement therapy, including increased risks for heart disease, breast cancer, and stroke. In fact, certain types of HRT have a higher risk than others, and the level of risk can vary from woman to woman depending upon her health history and lifestyle.

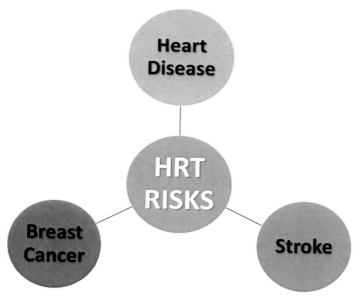

It is important to discuss both the risks and benefits with your doctor. Typically, the best route is to take the lowest dose and re-evaluate the treatment every six months.

The biggest study on this issue was the Women's Health Initiative mentioned above, which was a 15-year study that looked at more than 160,000 women who were past menopause.

According to the study, women who took both estrogen and progesterone had an increased chance of developing cardiovascular disease.

In the study, the risks of taking these medications over the long term outweighed any benefits taking the medication had on menopausal symptoms.

For some women, hormone replacement therapy is never appropriate. Talk to your healthcare provider if you have any of these conditions and are considering taking hormone replacement therapy:

- A history of blood clots, such as deep vein thrombosis or pulmonary emboli.
- A history of uterine, endometrial, or breast cancer
- A history of cardiovascular disease

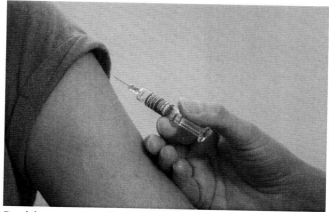

- Problems with liver disease in the past or present
- A previous heart attack
- Possible pregnancy
- History of stroke

If you have any of these conditions, the risk of taking hormone replacement therapy may outweigh the benefits of taking the therapy and there may be other medications that will be more beneficial.

Side Effects Of Hormone Replacement Therapy

There are side effects of taking hormone replacement therapy that may be significant enough that you may stop taking the medication or may not wish to start taking it. These include:

- Breast tenderness or swelling
- Bloating of the abdomen
- Changes in mood
- Nausea
- Headaches
- Vaginal bleeding

If you have any of these symptoms, talk to your doctor about whether or not hormone replacement therapy is right for you.

Weighing The Pros And Cons Of HRT

Read all you can about taking hormone replacement therapy and know your past and present medical history. Take this information to your doctor in order to decide if it is safe for you to take this type of therapy.

For some women, especially those with severe symptoms, it may be the only way to control the symptoms. If the symptoms are mild or there are other health issues to consider, hormone replacement may not be the best choice for you.

- Nicki had had it. At 49, she was just not feeling like herself. She was moody. One minute she felt on top of the world, the next, she felt like the world was going to overtake her, and the moment after that she felt like she wanted to kill someone. She found herself crying at TV commercials for what seemed like no reason. When she finally got to sleep at night, she'd awake in a pool of sweat or so hot she had to throw off the covers. She couldn't remember where she put her keys now, though she'd never lost anything before. Facts and names she always recalled just wouldn't come forward. During the day she was having a hot flash every 20 minutes and feeling like she just couldn't control her internal temperature. She went to her doctor and talked about the symptoms. She started HRT and the symptoms improved. She sleeps better and doesn't have all the mood swings. It's made a huge difference in her life.

- Alexandra had a partial hysterectomy 7 years ago and did not receive any HRT. She was 44 years old then and was fine for about 6 years but then experienced terrible headaches and once even passed out. Her doctors performed several costly tests that found nothing. Now at age 51, the hot flashes, incontinence, weight gain, and brittle hair convinced her doctor to prescribe Estradiol. After a little over week,

Alexandra's already experiencing fewer hot flashes and decreased bloating.

6 | Sexual Problems Associated With Menopause

A woman's libido is strongly associated with the amount of estrogen, progesterone, and testosterone she has in her body. As the levels of these hormones decrease, the sex drive will also decrease. This can affect her relationship with her sexual partner.

Estrogen is also important in having enough vaginal lubrication, and in the thickness and elasticity of the vaginal lining.

Without estrogen, there can be pain from intercourse associated with dryness of the vaginal mucosa. Fortunately, there are some remedies.

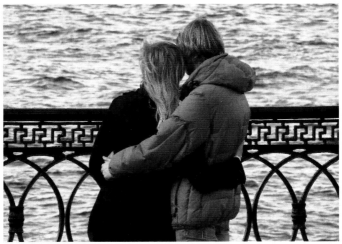

Hormone replacement therapy given orally or by any of the other acceptable routes can increase the thickness of the vaginal mucosa and prevent the dryness associated with menopause. For women who do not want to take a formal course of hormone replacement therapy, vaginal estrogen therapy can be provided.

Vaginal estrogen therapy is by prescription only. It can be administered in several ways, including creams, tablets, or a ring inserted into the vagina. These treatments provide local estrogen and do not appreciably increase the amount of estrogen in the bloodstream. Vaginal estrogen can increase the moisture in the vagina and decrease pain with intercourse.

For those women who do not want to use hormones, there are a variety of over-the-counter lubricants and moisturizers that can be used to make intercourse more comfortable. Some can be used on a regular basis, while others are used just prior to intercourse in order to lubricate the vaginal tissues.

7 | Health Risks Following Menopause

Menopause increases the risk of several diseases.

Heart Disease

As the estrogen level drops, the protective effect of estrogen on heart disease diminishes so that post-menopausal women begin to have a risk for heart disease that approaches that of men. They often get heart disease later in life when compared to men. As women age, the risk for heart disease, including heart attack, stroke, and peripheral vascular disease goes up.

Osteoporosis

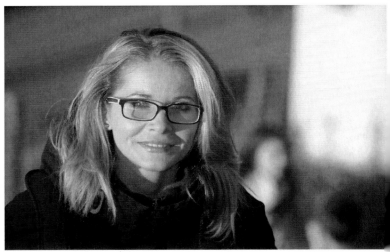

Women in menopause also have a risk for developing bone loss. Estrogen is required to keep calcium in the bones and without it, the calcium leaches out of the bones and the bones become thin. Mildly thinning bones is called osteopenia. Severely thinning bones is called osteoporosis.

Without the protective effect of estrogen, osteoporosis can result in vertebral fractures, particularly in the thoracic area. This results in the typical "dowager's hump" seen in women who have had compression of the vertebrae in the thoracic area of the spine.

The bones of the wrist and hip may also thin as a result of lowered estrogen levels. This causes an increased risk of fractures to each of these bones during a fall. When it comes to hip fractures, it is unclear as to whether the hip fractures prior to the fall or as a result of a minor fall. Either way, it can be very debilitating to suffer a fracture associated with osteoporosis, as the healing can be prolonged.

Stroke

Postmenopausal women have an increased risk of stroke. This is usually due to cholesterol and calcium building up in the carotid arteries. Clots can then form in these arteries, resulting in a stroke. There are medications that are prescribed for women (and men☺) with elevated cholesterol levels, which may reduce the risk of stroke.

Norma had been feeling great on hormone replacement. In fact, it helped so much she had stopped feeling like she wanted to kill someone every other minute. It was such a relief! The brain fog lifted and she started feeling more like herself. She also tried to eat healthier and get more exercise, but she just couldn't quit the cigarettes. She had cut down to just 4 day and felt like she was winning. When the headache started, she wasn't sure what was going on. Then her left arm wouldn't move when she told it to. Nothing felt right. She became confused but was able to call her son to take her to the hospital. Testing confirmed she'd had a mild stroke. With time and physical therapy she was able to regain the use of her arm. She finally was able to quit smoking, but unfortunately hormone replacement was no longer an option.

Peripheral Vascular Disease

The same is true of peripheral vascular disease. In peripheral vascular disease, however, the blood vessels affected are the arteries leading to the limbs, particularly the legs. Blood clots can form in the narrowed arteries, resulting in a loss of blood flow to the affected leg and a chance of developing gangrene of the leg. This may be treated by urgently removing the clot and expanding the size of the affected blood vessel.

Breast Cancer

Postmenopausal women have a greater risk of developing breast cancer, especially if they take unopposed estrogen (no progesterone) for their hot flashes. Up to 1 in 8 women will develop breast cancer sometime in their lives and the risk goes up with age.[15]

Regular mammograms can detect the presence of early breast cancer. Early detection and treatment are the keys to preventing advanced disease.

Dementia or Alzheimer's Disease

Estrogen may have an effect on a woman's cognition. The reasons for this are unclear. Postmenopausal women are at a greater risk of developing age-related dementia or Alzheimer's disease. Hormone replacement therapy may reduce the risk of these diseases.

---

[15] https://www.cancer.org/content/dam/cancer-org/research/cancer-facts-and-statistics/breast-cancer-facts-and-figures/breast-cancer-facts-and-figures-2017-2018.pdf

8 | Will This Ever End?

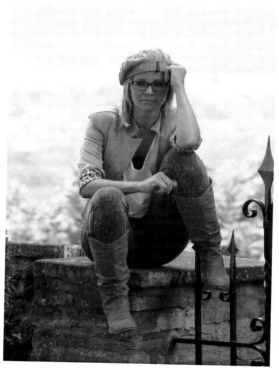

When you add up the years a woman is in perimenopause and the time she is in menopause, it can add up to as many as ten years with hot flashes, night sweats, mood swings, insomnia, and other menopausal symptoms.

Some women have no problems with menopause while others are severely afflicted with symptoms.

The best way to survive these years is to take good care of your body by exercising regularly, getting enough sleep, reducing stress, and eating a healthy diet.

If lifestyle factors are insufficient in controlling menopausal symptoms, things like herbal remedies for hot flashes or hormone replacement therapy may be necessary.

Talk to your healthcare provider about the best way to tackle the menopausal years and to get through the symptoms.

Eventually, the symptoms stop and you become post-menopausal, during which time the hormones are relatively stable, albeit much lower than before menopause.

9 | Finding Support and Getting Help

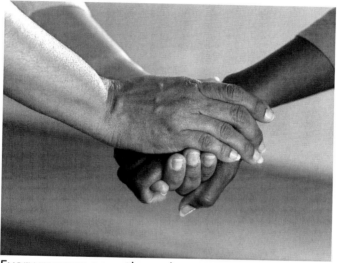

Every woman goes through menopause at some time during her life with the average age being 51 years of age. If you are suffering from severe symptoms, seek medical attention and discuss the various ways of coping with your symptoms.

Your healthcare provider may recommend herbal therapies, estrogen replacement therapy, or lifestyle changes in order to cope with the symptoms.

Our Menopause Movement Facebook group is a great place to get some of the support you need: https://www.facebook.com/groups/menopausemovement/

In the group, you can hear other women's stories, share your own, and find different ways of coping with the symptoms you are experiencing.

Conclusion

Menopause and perimenopause are facts of life and represent a major change in a woman's reproductive life and in her life in general. There may be months where the symptoms of menopause are nearly unbearable that are interspersed with months where the symptoms are not so bad.

The good news is that menopause can be conquered by any woman with the help of her healthcare professional and a group of like-minded women.

Through the use of lifestyle changes, hormone replacement therapy, and possibly herbal remedies, the symptoms of hot flashes, night sweats, insomnia, vaginal dryness, and mood swings can be overcome.

Be kind to yourself and practice self-care whenever possible, more than you have in your entire life. It is never selfish to make yourself a priority. Remember that when you are well, you are more equipped to take care of your loved ones.

> Do anything that helps improve your peace of mind, and quality of life.

Each woman's experience with menopause is unique to her. Your menopausal experience may be completely different from your siblings, friends, and neighbors.

This is why it is important to talk to your healthcare provider about your overall health as well as things you might be able to do (or not do) that can make the perimenopausal and menopausal years tolerable and improve your quality of life.

About the Author

Dr. Michelle Gordon believes in living life to the fullest. She has a passion for travel and has been to all the continents except Antarctica. That will be remedied in January of 2020. She is a board-certified general surgeon and founded Gordon Surgical Group in Putnam Valley, NY, in 2005.

She is the founder of Menopause Movement: A vibrant community of women helping women get through menopause. She founded Menopause Movement when she found herself in menopause and unable to find help (as a doctor!). Through comprehensive study, she transformed her menopause and her life. It is her mission to demystify menopause and help women understand this amazing stage in life.

In addition to the surgical practice, Michelle is enthusiastic about living a healthy and meaningful life. She is a fitness enthusiast and human diet advocate. She is a proponent of balanced, passionate living. When not traveling the world, she resides in Cortlandt Manor, NY, with her wife, Dr. Valerie Zarcone, and their two Newfoundlands, Sushi and Sashimi.

Manufactured by Amazon.ca
Acheson, AB